Herbal Medicine Cooker

The Best Solutions to Cook and Transform Herbs for Healing and Losing Weight

The information in the following pages is broadly considered a truthful and accurate account of facts and as such, any inattention, use, or misuse of the information in question by the reader will render any resulting actions solely under their purview. There are no scenarios in which the publisher or the original author of this work can be in any fashion deemed liable for any hardship or damages that may befall them after undertaking information described herein.

Additionally, the information in the following pages is intended only for informational purposes and should thus be thought of as universal. As befitting its nature, it is presented without assurance regarding its prolonged validity or interim quality. Trademarks that are mentioned are done without written consent and can in no way be considered an endorsement from the trademark holder.

Table of Contents

Chapter 1: Introduction

Welcome to the *Herbal Medicine Cooker*. You may be approaching this book as a practiced herbal healer, or you may simply be looking for a new weight loss technique. You might have a sense of what herbs can do for you, or you may just be starting to learn. Wherever you are in your life and your relationship with healing herbs, you've come to the right place.

This book applies ancient and modern scientific and spiritual knowledge about herbs to create recipes for meals that can better the lives of those who eat them. Whether you seek weight loss or better health in general, a return to herbal remedies through food may be exactly what you need to move forward.

Before we get to the recipes, however, we will discuss the history of herbal healing, how herbal healing works, the tools you'll need for this cooker, and then we'll go over which herbs have what benefit. When we get to those tasty recipes, you'll find three sections: cooked herbs, raw herbs, and steamed herbs. Each section has at least ten recipes for your delight.

You're on the path to healing, and you should be proud of yourself for taking your health into your own hands! By applying the knowledge in *Herbal Medicine Cooker* to your daily life, you're sure to succeed at your goals. Thank you for the download, and welcome to your future.

Chapter 2: Learning the Herbal Ways

History of Healing Herbs

Long before the Western world as we know it existed, long before ancient communities rose and fell in Greece and Rome, and long before even the pyramids in Egypt were constructed and abandoned, herbs were used for medicinal purposes. In the extent of written history, the presence of herbal healing exists, and even in times of prehistory, herbs were used to treat and mitigate ailments.

People have been using herbs as medicine all across history, writing down their practices and associations as they went. Today, we have that wealth of information to draw from when we begin our work of healing ourselves (and others) with herbs. From ancient Greece and Rome to China, India, Mesopotamia, Egypt, North, and South America, people in every continent on earth in every stage of history have uplifted herbs and minerals for their curative abilities. From those ancient times to today, the information remains the same, but it comes to *you* now for *your* own growth and well-being.

How Does It Work?

Ancient Romans used the herb dill to cleanse the air in their chambers. Ancient Greeks used laurel to crown victors and leaders. Prehistoric humans used herbs and drew them on the walls of their caves. But how did these people know that herbs would heal them? And how does the healing actually work?

Regardless of how these ancient peoples found out, they were definitely tapped into to something real that's actually backed by modern-day science. Essentially, all herbs and minerals have chemical compounds that, when consumed, become dispersed through the body of the eater. When your body takes in these chemicals, they fulfill needs that you likely weren't even conscious of having.

For those working toward weight loss, stick with herbs that are experts at inflammation reducing and metabolisms kick-starting such as **dandelion**, **cayenne pepper**, **goji berries**, **lemon & lemongrass**, **fenugreek**, and **psyllium**. For those working toward healing, literally every herb has something different to offer, so you'll have to do a little research into what herb works best for your ailment. A guide later in this cooker will likely help you with this effort.

Some techniques for herb preparation make them more effective as medicines. For example, grilling with herbs often chars them and removes any nutrition or healing potential. However, including rosemary with your grill marinade (or even a couple sprigs just set into the grill as you work) can help the nutrients of your meal remain intact. Roasting is not as bad as grilling but cooking on even a low heat for over 45 minutes starts to break down the nutrients left in your herbs and slightly lessen its healing potential. If you're going to be cooking with heat for this long, dried herbs are often a better way to go. For boiling and steaming, dry herbs work as well as fresh, for the bioavailability of fresh is mostly equivalent to dry herb, but it is true that the nutrition of fresh vastly outweighs that of dry.

Some herbs help to calm nausea while others release necessary vitamins. Some help with weight loss and may reduce inflammation generally. When it comes to herbs and their healing power, all you have to do is consume them, with varying degrees of prep involved. After one meal packed with healing herbs, you will easily and effortlessly assimilate nutrients, medicinal chemicals, and other bioavailable medicines into your body. Indeed, after you create a habit of eating like this, you'll find yourself getting better or shedding that weight in no time.

Gathering Your Tools

When you go to approach your new herb-infused diet for healing, you'll need a few things before you get started. First things first, you need an herbal connection. You'll really want to use fresh herbs whenever you're able to for a number of reasons. Mainly, your food will taste fresher, your herbs will be fuller of nutrients, and your meal will be overall healthier.

Eventually, growing your own herbs will be ideal, but even harvesting weekly bundles of fresh herbs from your local gardener, garden nursery, or garden store could work for now. You'll need some sort of fresh supply of herbs to start, clearly, but as you take those first steps, you can always just use any grocery store variety of pre-packaged fresh herbs.

When buying herbs, below are some hints of what to look for.

The Fresher, the Better

As mentioned above, fresher herbs have both a better taste and more bioavailable nutrients.

What to Avoid

Stay away from discolored herbs. If they're prepackaged and yellowing, there is likely some degree of rot somewhere in the packaging. Keep your herbs fresh and green.

Prep Your Herbs After Purchase

Especially when the herbs are prepackaged, you'll want to prep them for use once you've brought them home. Take the herbs out of their packaging and bundle them together with a rubber band or twist-tie. Once they're bundled together, snip off an inch or so from the base of their stems. Then, take a paper towel and wet it. You want it to be damp but not dripping wet. Wrap your herb stems in the paper towel and put it all in a plastic bag in your refrigerator until you're ready to use the herbs for cooking.

Wash Before Use

When you're ready to cook with those herbs, rinse them lightly before use and pick off any leaves that may have gone bad in the fridge. The prep techniques you used have helped to preserve the herbs for longer, but you may still have to pick away some bits. Shake the herbs dry as best you can and then use them however the recipe requires.

Furthermore, when it comes to the recipes in this cooker, you'll need a certain selection of tools. Here's a guide of what you can aim for:

Juicer

For the section on raw herbs, a juicer will be ideal to have, but if you don't have access to a juicer or the ability to get one, you can use a blender on its highest setting instead.

Herb Shears

If you've bought herbs in pots or if you're growing your own herbs in your garden, you'll need herb shears for harvest. Simply picking leaves off the plant can be traumatic to its overall survival, and those who are trying to keep the herb alive in their house or garden for years will want to be a little more respectful in their method of harvest. Herb shears allow you to carefully choose and the right leaves and only the ones you need. For that robust herbal flavor you want, snip off a handful of leaves, but always start from the outside of the plant or bundle and move to the inside. Furthermore, don't neglect the stems! They have as much flavor as the leaves sometimes, and other times, they can simply be useful to have intact for your recipe. Try snipping off whole stems from your herb plants, too.

Drying Devices

If you have your own fresh herbs – whether prepackaged from the store or from your own harvest – don't forget that you can also then dry them yourself! Although fresh herbs are preferred, you can always substitute for half the amount in dried herb form. Dried herbs at the store are incredibly expensive, however, and it's ideal to replace those herbal supplies once a year. That upkeep can get costly! Instead, you can dry your own herbs in several different ways, and that is a largely untapped potential for many herbal cookers.

You can use a dehydrator, a baking tray filled with fresh herbs set in the hot sun, or a baking sheet in the oven set at a low temperature. You can also try constructing your own drying "rack" with a regular triangular coat hanger and some twine. Simply tie three or four pieces of twine to the bottom rung of the hanger and then tie small bundles of fresh herbs to the bottom of each piece of twine. You can hang these herbs in your home or outside. It should only take a week for most herbs to fully dry with this method. Grind the dried herbs with a mortar and pestle or the butt of a knife before use. You could also simply chop them finely with a blade.

Multi-Cooker

For the section on cooked herbs, a multi-cooking appliance will be helpful to have, but if you don't have access to one, you can always use a variety of other kitchen pots and pans to make things work.

What Herb Does What?

Herb Name	Properties of Healing
Allspice	Anti-flatulent, anti-inflammatory, warming, heals the intestinal tract.
Basil	High in plant polyphenols, antibacterial, anti-inflammatory, may help with cancer, fights stress.
Bay Leaf	Helps immunity, provides sinus relief, treats arthritis.
Cardamom	Reduces bad breath and cavities, can treat infections and help with digestive troubles.
Cayenne Pepper	Weight loss agent (!), metabolism stimulator.
Chamomile	Lessens the likelihood of heart disease by increasing the sense of calm (among other things), full of antioxidants, helps with sleep.
Chili Powder	Boosts immunity, provides essential vitamins A, C, & E; reduces inflammation, pain, and sinus congestion.
Chives	Decreases risk of the stomach or digestion-related cancers.
Cilantro	Detoxifies, supports the heart, balances blood sugar, relieves anxiety, boosts your brain, and provides lots of vitamin A for vision.

Cinnamon	Encourages healthy skin, helps heal your brain, fights infection, works as an antioxidant, and fights brain degenerative diseases.
Cloves	Improves liver health, helps reduce ulcers, encourages bone strength, balances blood sugar, antibacterial.
Coriander	Provides lots of manganese, iron, and magnesium.
Cumin	Lots of vitamins help reverse damage done by hemorrhoids, general digestion aid, antioxidant abilities.
Curry Powder	Works against Alzheimer's disease degeneration, helps your heart, works against colon cancer.
Dandelion	Weight loss agent (!), increases metabolism, works as a diuretic and laxative, lowers cholesterol.
Dill	High in calcium and iron, anti-flatulent, lowers cholesterol, natural breath freshener, anti-cancer properties.
Echinacea	Incredibly powerful immunity booster.
Fennel Seed	Let go of excess water being retained in the body, cleanses the blood, and reduces symptoms of asthma, great for eyesight.

Fenugreek	Weight loss agent (!), reduces fat mass, lowers fever when present, heals kidneys and liver and relieves menstrual cramps.
Garlic	Protects against cancer, slows the progress of other illnesses, and reverses hypertension.
Ginger	Great for bellyache, anti-inflammatory, helps with diarrhea and nausea, high in good minerals.
Goji Berries	Weight loss agent (!), has anti-aging effects, lowers cholesterol, balances blood sugar, boosts energy naturally.
Hawthorne	Works as a natural flu shot, reverses congestive heart failure, helps with indigestion, lowers high blood pressure.
Lemon	Weight loss agent (!), hydrates exceedingly well, provides Vitamin C, heals the skin and freshen the breath, reverses kidney stones, helps digestion.
Lemongrass	Weight loss agent (!), burns fat and boosts metabolism, heals hair and skin, reverses cold and flu symptoms, relieves cramping pain during menses.
Lime	Benefits digestion, heart disease, and blood sugar; fights infections, cancer, and inflammation.

Marjoram	Diuretic, heals urinary tract, helps the release of toxins from the body, cleanses kidneys, and lowers blood pressure.
Mint/Peppermint	Works against Irritable Bowel Syndrome, encourages the flow of bile from the body, aids speed of digestion, calms tummy-ache.
Mustard Seed	Great source of selenium, omega-3 fatty acids, and manganese as well as vitamin B1, copper, magnesium, and phosphorous.
Nutmeg	Natural pain reliever, helps with sleeplessness, heals brain damage, works against bad breath, and promotes healthy skin and healthy circulation.
Oregano	Anti-inflammatory, rejects viral infections, high in antioxidants, might fight cancer, anti-bacterial.
Paprika	Prevents balding or hair loss, anti-inflammatory, decreases the threat of heart attack, can heal surface-level skin wounds.
Parsley	Lowers blood pressure, reduces hypertension, high in vitamin K among others, antifungal, antibacterial.

Psyllium	Probiotic, weight loss agent (!), speeds up the elimination of waste, reduces feelings of hunger. ** DO NOT USE IF PREGNANT OR ASTHMATIC **
Rosemary	Works toward overall heart health, lessen joint pain; boosts brain capacity, memory abilities, and cognitive functions.
Sage	Boosts brain power, increases memory retention and recall, anti-inflammatory, high in antioxidants.
St. John's Wort	May reverse Parkinson's disease, heals depression, helps with PMS, and reverses IBS, antiviral & antibacterial.
Stinging Nettle	Encourages hair health & growth, alleviate joint pain and reduces inflammation related to arthritis.
Tarragon	High in magnesium, iron, and zinc; use fresh leaves for best healing abilities, protects against the formation of dementia in the brain, defends stomach against worms and parasites.

Thyme	High in vitamin C, microbial, treat a sore throat, helps with tummy-ache, lessens pains of arthritis.
Turmeric	Reverses inflammation, high in antioxidants, most bioavailable when consumed with a dash of black pepper, boosts neuroplasticity.
Valerian	Encourages heart health, natural pain reliever, natural muscle relaxant, natural sleep aid, relieves anxiety.

Chapter 3: The Recipes

Some of the recipes in this book are vegan, some are gluten-free, and some are filled with cheese and meat. Whatever your dietary inclination is, however, this book can work for you. No matter what the recipe base is — whether raw vegan or cooked & meaty or anything in between — there will always be room for alternatives to suit your dietary needs. Herbal healing isn't exclusive to any one diet, in particular, so you can always make these recipes work for you while retaining that healing potential.

Additionally, the recipes in this book range from longer to shorter, more intensive or less — but none of them are incredibly complicated. You will always be warned when you need a kitchen appliance, and you will often have alternatives suggested based on a number of dietary restrictions, in case you happen to have any.

You are always invited to add more of any spice or herb that you desire, especially for the first batch of recipes, for any dilution of flavor through heat (or otherwise) can be remedied simply by adding just a touch (or so) more. Overall, in this chapter, you will be guided through your experience with herbal healing one recipe at a time, beginning with the stews, so let's heat it up and get started.

Cooking with Herbs – Soups & Stews

From soups to stews and heated aromatherapy, this section focuses on bringing your herbs past the boiling point. Some of the recipes require simmering for longer than 45 minutes, and in that case, you could use dried or fresh herbs for those creations. Otherwise, try to keep your recipes dedicated to the preservation and display of *fresh* herbs whenever possible. You'll be grateful you did so, trust me.

Mussels & Clams with Herbs de Provence

This recipe won't take your herbs past their boiling point too much, so you can feel free to amp it up with the freshest of ingredients for this recipe (unless otherwise noted). If you're vegetarian or vegan, you can still try this recipe with just mussels; they have no central nervous system and don't feel pain! Decide as you will, however. It'll surely be delicious for those who try.

This recipe needs 15 minutes of prep and 20 minutes of cooking. It will make 6 helpings.

What to Use:

- Onion (1 medium-sized, chopped small)
- Garlic (3 cloves, minced)
- Olive Oil (1 tablespoon)
- Diced Tomatoes (1 16-ounce can, undrained)
- White Wine (1 cup, dry white wine preferred)
- Tomato Paste (1.5 teaspoons)
- Mushrooms (1 handful of any variety, sliced thinly)
- Basil (0.25 cup fresh herb)
- Oregano (2 sprigs fresh herb)
- Tarragon (0.25 cup fresh herb)

- Thyme (2 sprigs fresh herb)
- Parsley (1 tablespoon *dried* herb)
- Marjoram (1 tablespoon *dried* herb)
- Rosemary (2 springs fresh herb)
- Fennel Seed (1 tablespoon)
- Mussels (1 pound, washed & scrubbed)
- Clams (1 pound, washed & scrubbed)
- Olives (0.5 cup, any variety)
- Tomatoes (2 fresh medium-sized, chopped small)
- Fettuccini Pasta (12 ounces, precooked) OR French Bread (1 or more baguettes, cut into slices and toasted)
- 1 large pot (only used to cook your pasta if you choose to serve with pasta) & 1 large saucepan

What to Do:

- With the olive oil added to your saucepan on a medium-high heat, cook the onion and garlic for about 5 minutes.
- Add in the canned diced tomatoes, wine, and tomato paste and bring to a low boil.
- Separately, get all your herbs prepared. If you have a tea ball, stuff as many herbs as you can into that ball, but if not, that's going to be fine.

- Stir the mushrooms, mussels, and clams into the pan and then add your spices. If you're using the tea ball, go ahead and plop it in. If you're just placing your herbs into the pan, bundle together the sprigs of rosemary, oregano, and thyme so that they're easier to remove at the end. Chop the other herbs finely in this case before adding them to the pan.
- Cover the pan. Simmer under low heat for 10 minutes or until all mussels and clams have opened and mushrooms are perfectly tender.
- Remove lid and add olives and fresh tomatoes. Cover once more and simmer for 5 minutes.
- Serve with fresh bread or with pasta.

Pot Roast for Your Heart

This pot roast is focused on rosemary to help heal your heart. While pot roast does use red meat, which isn't great for those with heart issues, the spices involved can do a lot to boost your health despite that aforementioned complication. Grab your multi-cooker or slow-cooker for this one and get ready for a delicious meal later!

This recipe needs 15 minutes of prep and up to 10 hours of cooking. It will make 6 helpings.

What to Use:

- Beef Chuck Roast (2 pounds of boneless meat, cubed)
  - For vegetarian or vegan substitution, try 4 pounds of a variety of mushrooms!
- Potatoes (3 medium-sized, cubed)
- Carrots (2 large, sliced)
- Celery (2 stalks, sliced)
- Onion (1 large-sized, chopped)
- Diced Tomatoes (1 16-ounce can, undrained)
- Cream of Mushroom Soup (1 12-ounce can)
  - Vegan alternatives exist!
- Water (0.5 cup)
- Tomato Paste (2 tablespoons)

- Rosemary (1 teaspoon *dried* herb & 2 sprigs fresh herb)
- Salt (0.5 teaspoon)
- 1 multi-cooker

What to Do:

- Prepare your beef chunks, herbs, and veggies first. For the rosemary on sprigs, grab the base of the sprig and pull back to get all the leaves off the stems and then chop the fresh leaves roughly. Discard the stems.
- Then grab your multi-cooker or slow-cooker. Spray the inside lightly with cooking spray, then add potatoes and onions into the pot to cook first.
- Over the potatoes and onions, lay the celery, carrots, and beef in that order. Then you can add all the remaining ingredients at once.
- Use the cooker on a high setting for 5 hours or on low for 10. Cook as needed until beef is tender then serve!

Homestyle Brain-Boosting Gravy

Using such iconic herbs as parsley, sage, rosemary, and thyme, this gravy is full of brain-boosting potential. It's delicious, nutritious, and absolutely bursting with healing abilities. Serve with whatever you like, whether it's a cold turkey sandwich or freshly cooked veggies.

This recipe needs 5 minutes of prep and an hour and a half of cooking. It will make 2 helpings.

What to Use:

- Potatoes (2 medium-sized)
- Button Mushrooms (2 handfuls)
- Carrots (3 medium-sized, cut in chunks)
- Celery (3 stalks, cut in chunks)
- Onion (1 small-sized, cut into eight pieces)
- Garlic (3 cloves, smashed)
- Olive Oil (1 tablespoon)
- Red Wine (0.25 cup, dry red wine preferred)
- Tomato Paste (1 tablespoon)
- Parsley (4 fresh sprigs)
- Thyme (4 fresh sprigs)
- Rosemary (4 fresh sprigs)
- Marjoram (2 fresh sprigs)
- Sage (2 fresh sprigs)
- Bay Leaf (2)

- Peppercorns (12)
- 1 large Dutch oven
- 1 blender or immersion blender

What to Do:

- With the oven preheated to 425 degrees F, cut one of your potatoes into quarters and heat it up in a large Dutch oven with the mushrooms and remaining vegetables. Add the olive oil and stir to coat.
- Roast for 30 minutes like this, stirring every 10 minutes. Vegetables will become deeply browned on edges.
- Pull the Dutch oven from the oven and bring it to the stove top. Pour in the wine and tomato paste then add 8 cups of water. Add all the remaining ingredients and stir.
- On high heat, bring the Dutch oven to a boil then without a lid, simmer for 30 minutes. Once the timer is up, let the mixture stand for 10 minutes.
- Strain out the liquid and keep it in a separate bowl. Discard the solid ingredients from the Dutch oven then pour the liquid back into the pot.
- Separately, prepare the other potato by peeling it and cutting into a small dice. Boil in the liquid for about 5 minutes then

simmer without a lid for 30. You want the water to be reduced into about 2.5 cups worth.

- As a final step, use an immersion blender to make smooth or pour everything from the pot into a blender and pulse until smooth.
- Strain as desired to remove chunks and season with salt and pepper as desired. Reheat if needed and serve.

Roasted Tomato Soup

This simple tomato soup is backed with the ability to protect against cancer, to boost your immunity, and to help reduce inflammation in your body. It will be a family favorite in no time, if not for its awesome effects then for its ease to make and delicious taste.

This recipe needs 25 minutes of prep and 1 hour of cooking. It will make 6 helpings.

What to Use:

- Tomatoes (5 pounds large-sized tomatoes, quartered & seeded)
- Olive Oil (0.33 cup)
- Garlic (8 cloves, minced)
- Onion (1 large-sized, chopped roughly)
- Water (2 cups)
- Salt (1 teaspoon)
- Black Pepper (0.33 teaspoon)
- Rosemary (1 teaspoon, *dried* herb)
- Thyme (1 teaspoon, *dried* herb)
- Sage (0.75 teaspoon, *dried* herb)
- Heavy Cream (0.5 cup – any unsweetened "mylk" alternative will do!)
- Basil (1 cup fresh leaves, chopped for garnish)
- Red Pepper Flakes (for garnish, optional)

- 1 baking sheet for broiling
- 1 large pot
- 1 blender or immersion blender

What to Do:

- With the oven preheated to 400 degrees F, grease your baking sheet and line it with your prepped tomatoes. Drizzle with oil and minced garlic. Toss lightly to coat.
- Bake 20 minutes until soft, stirring a few times in the process.
- Pull from oven and remove skins. Discard them, for we won't need them.
- In a large pot, sauté the cut onion with a dash of oil, then add your tomatoes with the water and spices up to the sage. Boil and reduce heat to simmer.
- Cook 30 minutes until flavors are well-combined. Use an immersion blender to smooth mix or pour out batches into a blender and pulse until smooth.
- Eventually, all the soup should be completely smooth and returned to the pot to be heated through. At this point, add the cream or mylk.
- Serve with garnish, as desired.

Lemon Fennel Soup

This raw soup requires few ingredients and really packs quite the punch. It will help you to detox and focus with its refreshing taste, and it will even clear out deep toxins like cancer through its simple profile and huge potential.

This recipe needs 5 minutes of prep and requires no cooking. It will make 4 helpings.

What to Use:

- Lemons (2, juiced)
- Water (3 cups)
- Extra Virgin Olive Oil (0.5 cup)
- Salt (1.5 teaspoons)
- Garlic (2 cloves, minced)
- Fennel Bulb (about 0.5 pound, sliced thinly)
- Scallions (2 stalks, sliced thinly)
- 4 bowls

What to Do:

- Whisk together the first five ingredients. They are our simple soup's base, and you can portion it out into fourths and pour them into each of the four bowls.

- Slice your fennel and scallions. Top the broth base with the sliced veggies and serve as is!
- This delightful and light soup will keep for about three days.

Kabobs with Herb Marinade

Whether you make this marinade with chicken, pork, beef, lamp, or simply veggies, you're bound to love its flavor and healing potential. If you have digestive issues normally, try this recipe on for size – it's well-suited to calm that tummy while making it feel warm and full.

This recipe needs 5 minutes of prep and 10 minutes of cooking. It will make 4 helpings.

What to Use:

- Chicken/Beef/Lamb/Pork/Veggies (1 pound, cut into inch-sized pieces)
- Olive Oil (3 tablespoons)
- Garlic (3 cloves, minced)
- Balsamic Vinegar (1 tablespoon)
- Lemon Juice (1 tablespoon)
- Oregano (1 tablespoon fresh herb)
- Cumin (0.5 teaspoon, *dried* herb)
- Basil (0.5 teaspoon, *dried* herb)
- Onion Powder (0.5 teaspoon)
- Sugar (0.5 teaspoon)
- Salt (0.5 teaspoon)
- Black Pepper (0.25 teaspoon)
- Paprika (0.25 teaspoon)
- 4 skewers (or use the rosemary sprigs *as* your skewers!)

- 1 small-sized bowl
- 1 large plastic bag
- 1 grill or sauté pan for grilling the kabobs

What to Do:

- Cut up your vehicle for the sauce, whether it's meat or veggie-based.
- Separately, stir together the marinade ingredients with a fork in a small-sized bowl and then pour it into the plastic bag.
- Add your meat or veg to the bag and toss everything with the bag sealed to coat.
- Marinate in the fridge for up to 8 hours.
- Let sit at room temperature for 10 minutes before assembling in skewers and attempting to grill.
- Cook on grill or in sauté pan on high heat for 5 minutes on each side until done to your preference!

Vitamin-Rich Root Soup

Full of essential vitamins and antioxidants, this soup will impress you with its healing abilities and its intense flavor. It's complex and well-rounded. It's a beautiful color to boot! You won't be able to get enough of this fall-time soup for sure, and you'll come back for more when you realize all it's doing for you on the inside, too.

This recipe needs 10 minutes of prep and 40 minutes of cooking. It will make 4 helpings.

What to Use:

- Coconut Oil (1.5 tablespoons)
- Sweet Onion (1 medium-sized, chopped)
- Garlic (2 cloves, minced)
- Ginger (1 inch of root, grated)
- Cumin (1 teaspoon)
- Coriander (1 teaspoon)
- Cinnamon (0.5 teaspoon)
- Nutmeg (0.5 teaspoon)
- Cardamom (0.5 teaspoon)
- Cayenne Pepper (0.25-0.5 teaspoon)
- Butternut Squash (1 small-sized, peeled & chopped)
- Sweet Potato (1 medium-sized, peeled & chopped)
- Carrots (2 medium-sized, peeled & sliced)

- Vegetable Broth (6-8 cups)
- Full-Fat Coconut Milk (1 14-ounce can)
- Salt & Pepper (to taste)
- Lemon (1, juiced for garnish)
- Cilantro (for garnish, fresh herb)
- 1 large-sized pot
- 1 blender or immersion blender

What to Do:

- Start by heating up the oil in your large pot on a low heat. Add in the onion and cook for about 5 minutes. Then add in the garlic and ginger and stir constantly for another minute.
- Add all the spices and sauté on medium heat for 2 minutes. If things start sticking to the pan, use a bit of broth to help it become unstuck.
- Now add the squash, sweet potato, and carrots. Sauté for 5 minutes and then pour in veggie broth.
- Bring the mix to high heat and boil before reducing to simmer. Cover before cooking 20 minutes.
- After 20 minutes, make sure vegetables are soft before adding coconut milk. Simmer 10 more minutes.

- After everything is well-cooked, use an immersion blender to make smooth or add in small batches to a blender until the whole batch of soup is perfectly smooth.
- Heat again as needed. As a final step, stir in the lemon juice and serve with cilantro as garnish.

Healing Chicken Soup from China

This ancient Chinese soup may use some herbs you've never heard of, but one trip to the right store can remedy that, and the *remedy* this soup makes is unheard of! It boosts immunity, prevents the flu and colds, and supposedly establishes a balance between your yin and yang energy!

This recipe needs 15 minutes of prep and up to four hours of cooking. It will make 4 helpings.

What to Use:

- Chicken (1 small-sized, about 3 pounds)
- Astragalus or *Huang Qi* (a root-like herb, 3 shoots)
- Dried Longan or *Long Yan Rou* (a handful of dried berries)
- Red Dates or *Hong Zoo* (a handful of pitted dates)
- Codonopsis or *Dang Shen* (like a dried bean, 5 "beans")
- Chinese Wild Yam or *Huai Shan* (0.5 cup)
- Goji Berries or *Gou Qi* (0.25 cup dried berries)
- Carrots (1.5 pounds, sliced)
- Ginger (1 inch of root, sliced)
- Salt (to taste)
- 1 large pot about half-full of water

What to Do:

- With your large pot that's half-full of water, parboil your chicken. Once it's boiling, let the chicken cook for 5 minutes. Remove chicken and thoroughly rinse.
- While this is boiling, rinse your herbs and let them sit to dry.
- Prepare your carrots and ginger and put them aside.
- When the chicken's done, take it out of the pot and dump the water from the pot. Fill it again with 8 cups of water, replace the chicken into the pot and add all other ingredients except salt.
- Bring to a boil and then simmer covered for up to 4 hours, stirring occasionally.
- Season with salt and serve!

Soulful Thai Stew

This spicy and warming soup is great for the winter months as well as the flu season. Traditionally called *Tom Kha*, this soup originates from Thailand with many different variations in existence today. With the fish sauce in this recipe, it might be hard to make vegetarian or vegan, but substitutions still exist! For these cases, try 2 tablespoons of maple syrup and a tablespoon of liquid aminos instead! This recipe is fresh and fiery, and it's sure to give you the strength and motivation needed to fight the cold, both literally and figuratively.

This recipe needs 5 minutes of prep and an hour and 35 minutes of cooking. It will make 10 helpings.

What to Use:

- Bone Broth (32 ounces or 4 cups)
- Coconut Milk (3 15-ounce cans)
- Lemongrass (2 big stalks, sliced into large chunks)
- Fish Sauce (4 tablespoons)
- Tamari (2 tablespoons)
- Apple Cider Vinegar (2 tablespoons)
- Lime Juice (4 tablespoons)
- Ginger (2 inches of root, minced)
- Garlic (8 cloves, minced)

- Chicken Thighs (1 pack – about 12 ounces, sliced)
- Shitake Mushrooms (1 cup, sliced)
- Bok Choy (1 bunch, chopped)
- Kale (1 bunch, chopped)
- Green Onions (1 bunch, sliced)
- Carrots (2 medium-sized, chopped)
- Thai Green Curry Paste (1 tablespoon)
- Cilantro (1 bunch fresh herb, chopped with stems)
- 1 large-sized pot

What to Do:

- In your large pot, bring to heat the bone broth and coconut milk. Just as the liquids come to a boil, add the fish sauce and tamari. Then stir in your apple cider vinegar, lime juice, ginger, and garlic.
- Simmer on low heat for 10 minutes.
- Add the chicken, mushrooms, greens, green onions, and carrots to the broth mixture. Stir and cook for a minute before adding the green curry paste.
- Cover and simmer for 20 minutes. Once the chicken is cooked completely, add the fresh cilantro and serve.

Herbal Stew from Persia

Traditionally called *Ghormeh Sabzi*, this herbed stew is a classic of Persian cuisine. Literally translated into cooked herbs, this stew is meant to be fragrant, filling, and satisfying, and it certainly won't disappoint! Serve it with mushrooms instead of meat to make it vegan or vegetarian, and don't forget to make yourself a side of rice for the most authentic experience possible.

This recipe needs 20 minutes of prep and two hours and 45 minutes of cooking. It will make 6 helpings.

What to Use:

- Parsley (4 bunches fresh herb)
- Cilantro (3 bunches fresh herb)
- Chives (2 bunches fresh herb)
- Fenugreek (1 bunch fresh herb or 1 tablespoon dried leaves)
- Vegetable Oil (0.5 cup)
- Yellow Onion (1 small-sized, diced)
- Beef or Lamb or Mushroom (1.5 pounds of meat or 2 pounds of mushrooms)
- Turmeric (1 teaspoon)
- Water (5 cups)
- Persian Dried Limes (also called *limoo amani*, soaked in water for an hour)
- Salt & Pepper (to taste)
- Kidney Beans (1 15-ounce can, drained)

- 1 large sauté pan
- Rice (precooked to serve with the stew)

What to Do:

- First, wash your fresh herbs, pat them dry, and chop them incredibly finely. You can use a food processor carefully if you'd rather not chop.
- In a large sauté pan on low heat, warm up a third-cup of oil and sauté your herbs for 10 minutes. You want them to dry out a little bit more. Then, add the remaining oil and sauté 15 minutes longer. Remove herbs from pan.
- Then, in the same pan, add a dash of oil and cook your onion on medium heat till translucent. Add in meat or mushrooms and your turmeric.
- Stir and sauté until the color becomes light brown in the pan before adding your water. Turn up the heat and bring to a boil. Reduce to simmer, covered, for 30 minutes.
- After 30 minutes, add your herbs back to the pan and cover. On the lowest heat, cook an hour to 1.5 hours. Meanwhile, soak your Persian dried limes.
- When ready, stick the limes with a fork and add them to the stew. Cook 15 minutes longer and serve with a scoop of rice.

DIY Healing Aromas

Did you know that you can make your own scent diffuser with just a pot, some herbs, and some water? Truly! You don't need essential oils or a fancy diffuser to get the benefits of herbal healing in the atmosphere of your home. Simply follow the instructions below to reap the benefits.

This recipe needs 0 minutes of prep and as many minutes of cooking as you like. It creates a scent concoction, so there really aren't "servings" for this recipe. Whoever's in the room or the floor of the house will be affected positively by the aromas.

What to Use:

- Water (6-8 cups)
- Herbs (whichever ones you desire; whether in combination or alone, fresh or dried)
- 1 medium-sized pot

What to Do:

- Bring the water in your pot to a boil and then add your herbs. Turn the heat down to medium-high and let boil, adding more water as needed and more herbs as needed to keep the scents diffusing.

- Refresh as needed and boil as long as desired to keep the scents billowing throughout your space.

Using Raw Herbs – Salads & Juices

In this section, we keep things a little cooler than the last. The aim here is to keep your herbal selection as close to raw as possible to retain those nutrients and healing aspects. You'll need a juicer or a blender for half of these recipes, but the other half often doesn't even require a sauté pan. Once again, you'll want to have fresh herbs whenever possible, especially when you approach the juices in the second half of this section. If you don't have fresh herbs for the juices, don't attempt them yet – it really won't be the same. With the salads, however, you might be able to get away with the dried herb in some cases. As always, do what you can, but fresh is always preferred.

Tabouli Salad

This refreshing take on traditional tabouli amps it up a notch with the help of allspice, cinnamon, and a good bit of mint. Feel free to swap out the bulgur for brown rice, white rice, pasta, or whatever else makes the herbs in this dish manageable for you to eat. Remember – it's all about the herbs in this cooker! Everything else around it can be interchanged and alternated or substituted as you desire.

This recipe needs 30 minutes of prep and assembly. It will make 6 helpings.

What to Use:

- Bulgur Wheat (0.25 cup)
- Water (2 cups, boiling)
- Parsley (30 ounces or 3.5 cups at least, destemmed, washed well, & chopped roughly)
- Mint (2.5 packed cups, chopped roughly)
- Tomatoes (5 medium-sized, diced finely)
- Onion (0.5 of a medium-sized onion, diced finely)
- Extra Virgin Olive Oil (0.5 cup)
- Lemon (1, juiced & zested)
- Paprika (0.5 teaspoon)
- Allspice (0.125 teaspoon ground & dried seed)

- Cinnamon (0.125 teaspoon ground herb)
- Salt (to taste)
- 1 medium-sized bowl
- 1 food processor

What to Do:

- In your small bowl, pour your bulgur and let sit as you boil the water. Eventually, pour the water into the bowl and cover for 20 minutes as the bulgur cooks itself. After 20 minutes, drain the wheat well and set it aside.
- Now, use your food processor to pulse together the remaining ingredients. Start with the parsley and mint and combine them well (without making them into an herbal mush) before adding the rest.
- Pour out your mixture into the medium-sized bowl with the bulgur and stir well to coat completely. Season with salt as desired and enjoy!

Pesto Pasta Salad

Need a chilled pasta salad to impress the family or friends for the reunion or upcoming party? Here's a go-to for just that occasion. Made with a refreshing vegan pesto (to which you can surely add cheese, as desired!), this pasta salad is all about undeniable, drool-inducing flavor. Once you have a bite, I think you'll get what I mean.

This recipe needs 5 minutes of prep and up to 25 minutes of cooking. It will make 4 helpings.

What to Use:

- Garlic (2 cloves)
- Salt (1 teaspoon)
- Pistachios (2 cups, deshelled)
- Basil (4 packed cups)
- Limes (3, juiced)
- Extra Virgin Olive Oil (0.5 cup)
- 1 blender
- Whole Grain Pasta (16 ounces)
- Red Pepper (0.5 of a medium-sized pepper, diced finely)
- Yellow Onion (0.5 of a medium-sized onion, diced finely)
- Kalamata Olives (0.5 cup, pitted & sliced)
- Artichoke Hearts (0.75 cup, chopped roughly)
- Raisins (0.33 cup)
- Peas (10 ounces, frozen & cooked)

- Chicken (precooked & shredded, if desired)
- Bacon (precooked & chopped, if desired)
- Up to 2 medium-sized pots
- 1 large-sized bowl

What to Do:

- Prepare the pesto first. In a blender, combine all the ingredients up until and including your extra virgin olive oil. If you need any extra liquid, feel free to juice an additional lime or two, or just add extra water or oil, based on the taste you're looking for. Pour the pesto into your large-sized bowl and move on.
- Separately, prepare your pasta in a medium-sized pot with enough water and boil until it's al dente.
- While the pasta's cooking, prepare the veggies for your pasta salad. Prep the pepper, onion, olives, artichoke hearts, and peas. For those peas, you'll use the second medium-sized pot to boil them from frozen to ready to eat.
- Once the pasta and peas are done, drain them and rinse them thoroughly with cool water.
- Mix everything together in the large bowl when the desired coolness is achieved. Stir well and enjoy!

Potato, Green Bean & Dill Salad

When green beans come into season in the summer, this recipe is the most delicious. Try to align it with the harvest of your dill for an incredible taste you'll come back for almost weekly. I swear – this recipe is addicting. Chefs beware! You'll love it so much, you won't be able to stop making it.

This recipe needs 5 minutes of prep and 15 minutes of cooking. It will make 4 helpings.

What to Use:

- Red Potatoes (12 ounces, small red potatoes, cut into quarter-inch-thick slices)
- Green Beans (12 ounces)
- Olive Oil (2 tablespoons)
- White Wine Vinegar (2 tablespoons)
- Dijon Mustard (1 tablespoon)
- Salt (0.5 teaspoon)
- Garlic Powder (0.25 teaspoon)
- Dill (0.5 teaspoon *dried* herb or 2 stalks fresh herb, chopped finely)
- Black Pepper (0.5 teaspoon)
- 1 medium-sized pot
- 1 medium-sized bowl
- 1 small-sized bowl

What to Do:

- Prepare your potatoes and then put them in your medium-sized pot with the green beans and about 6-8 cups of water to cover them. Turn the heat to high and boil for 2-3 minutes. Reduce the heat and simmer without a cover for 20 minutes longer, or until potatoes are completely tender.
- In a small separate bowl, mix together the olive oil, vinegar, mustard, salt, garlic, dill, and black pepper. This will be your dressing, and dang is it delicious.
- Once the potatoes and green beans are done, drain the liquid from them and put them into your medium-sized bowl. Pour the dressing on top and serve hot or chill for up to 2 hours before serving.

Thai Salad

This salad can calm tough tummy issues as well as provide a delicious and refreshing meal. You'll definitely want the freshest herbs for this recipe so that it heals to its fullest potential. If desired, you can always substitute the mung bean sprouts for some brown or white rice.

This recipe needs 10 minutes of prep and 5 minutes of assembly. It will make 4 helpings.

What to Use:

- Spinach (4 packed cups, cut or torn into one-inch pieces)
- Green Cabbage (0.25 head of cabbage, cored & sliced)
- Mint (1 packed cup, washed well & torn)
- Basil (1 packed cup, washed well & torn)
- Mung Bean Sprouts (2 cups)
- 1 large-sized bowl
- Kaffir Lime Leaves (6)
- Extra Virgin Olive Oil (1 cup)
- Lemon (0.5, juiced & zested)
- Nama Shoyu (1 tablespoon)
- Celery (2 stalks)
- Ginger (one half-inch of the root, grated)
- 1 blender

What to Do:

- Prepare your vegetables for the salad part and mix them together in your large bowl.
- Separately, combine the remaining ingredients in the blender and process until smooth. This mixture will be your dressing.
- Pour the dressing over your salad for a delightfully zippy South Asian salad experience.

Spring Herb & Dandelion Salad

This raw salad is made for your health. It's full of nutrients, minerals, and herbs that will inherently boost your automatic processes of digestion, respiration, and toxin-expelling. You'll soon find it a springtime and summertime favorite.

This recipe needs 10 minutes of prep and 5 minutes of assembly. It will make 4 helpings.

What to Use:

- Rainbow Chard (0.5 bunch, destemmed of toughest parts, cut into one-inch pieces)
- Red Cabbage (0.25 head of cabbage, cored & sliced thinly)
- Dill (1 bunch fresh herb, chopped roughly with stems)
- Rosemary (1 bunch fresh herb, destemmed & chopped roughly)
- Cilantro (0.5 bunch fresh herb, chopped roughly with stems)
- Dandelions (1-2 handfuls, chopped roughly)
    - o ** Make sure they're gathered from a yard that's not treated with pesticides or herbicides!!! **
- 1 large-sized bowl
- Curry Powder (1 tablespoon)

- Apple (1 medium-sized; halved, cored & diced)
- Garlic (2 cloves, minced)
- Ginger (one half-inch of the root, minced)
- Extra Virgin Olive Oil (1 cup)
- Lemon (1, juiced & zested)
- Salt (to taste)
- 1 blender

What to Do:

- Prepare the chard, cabbage, dill, rosemary, cilantro, and dandelions and place them into your large bowl.
- Put the next set of ingredients together in the blender and pulse until smooth to make your dressing.
- Pour dressing over your salad ingredients and enjoy a raw blast of herbal healing power!

Healing Green Juice

If you're low on necessary minerals in your diet or in your search for health, this juice may be the first place to start. This Healing Green Juice is full of vitamins and essential minerals as well as fiber and healthy sugars, not to mention those herbs! This recipe seeks to heal the heart, the blood, and the body as a whole. It's antifungal, antibacterial, anti-inflammatory, and it even works as a diuretic.

This recipe needs less than 5 minutes of prep to be ready! It will make up to 4 helpings, depending on how much you can drink.

What to Use:

- Spinach (2 packed cups, washed)
- Cucumbers (1 small-sized)
- Celery (2 stalks)
- Green Apple (1 large, cut into quarters & deseeded)
- Parsley (1 bunch, washed well)
- 1 juicer (or blender if absolutely impossible to get a juicer)

What to Do:

- If you have a juicer, add everything into your juicer, process, and drink as soon as possible. Make sure to put your greens in between two big pieces of something else otherwise they might not be able to be fully juiced. I like to stick the parsley bunch between pieces of apples so I'm sure it really gets processed.

- If you're using a blender, add a half-cup of water to your recipe and add more water as needed to get your blender going. Serve chilled!

"The Cure"

Now, this recipe doesn't taste the *greatest*, but one of the produce suppliers at my work swears to me he's cured someone's cancer with this drink. He prescribed it to a colleague – drink this concoction daily and just wait to see what happens! Their cancer was cured, and it may not happen for you, but it's worth a try! A blender works just fine for this recipe.

This recipe needs less than 5 minutes of prep to be ready! It will make up to 4 helpings, depending on how much you can drink.

What to Use:

- Lemon (1, rind & all)
- Parsley (2 bunches, washed well)
- Water (1-1.5 cups)
- Ginger (1.5 inches of root)
- Ice (1 small-sized handful)
- 1 blender (a juicer could work, too)

What to Do:

- Blend everything up at once. Depending on the speed and power of your blender, start with the water, ice, and greens and pulse until completely smooth before adding the chunkier bits.

- Enjoy chilled! (Plug your nose if needed or add a touch of agave nectar – I promise, your body wants this drink so badly!)

Detox Juice

This juice, when drunk daily, will help you absolutely flush your system. It'll push out toxins like the plague and make way in your system for only goodness and growth. The taste is complex and just a touch sweet.

This recipe needs less than 5 minutes of prep to be ready! It will make up to 4 helpings, depending on how much you can drink.

What to Use:

- Carrot (1 large-sized)
- Watermelon (1-2 large slices)
- Cucumber (1 medium-sized)
- Stinging Nettles (0.5 packed cup, washed well)
    - ** It may seem scary, but you can absolutely eat raw stinging nettles. As long as their leaves are broken down, they won't be able to "sting" you. You're safe when they're juiced or blended! **
- Cilantro (0.5 packed cup, washed well)
- Parsley (0.25 packed cup, washed well)
- 1 juicer (or 1 blender could work, too)

What to Do:

- If you have a juicer, add everything into your juicer, process, and drink as soon as possible. Make sure to put your nettle, parsley, and cilantro greens in between two big pieces of something else otherwise they might not be able to be fully juiced.
- If you're using a blender, add a half-cup of water to your recipe, ditch the watermelon rind, cut everything into much smaller pieces, and add more water as needed to get your blender going. Serve chilled!

Mood-Booster Juice

If you've been struggling with low mood, this might be the juice for you. It can help combat depression as well as low motivation and lack of ambition. Go to this juice when you're feeling down in the dumps. Its gorgeous color is sure to cheer you up if nothing else!

This recipe needs less than 5 minutes of prep to be ready! It will make up to 4 helpings, depending on how much you can drink.

What to Use:

- Beet (1 large, quartered)
- Spinach (2 packed cups, washed well)
- Apple (1 large, quartered & deseeded)
- Carrot (1 large)
- Turmeric (1 inch of root)
- St. John's Wort (1 tablespoon *dried* herb, stirred in at the end)
- Black Pepper (a dash at the end)
- 1 juicer (or 1 blender could work, too)

What to Do:

- If you have a juicer, add everything into your juicer, process, and drink as soon as possible. Make sure to sprinkle and stir in your St. John's Wort & black pepper before consuming! That herb is a powerful mood-booster you won't want to miss, and the black pepper is pivotal in making the abilities of the turmeric root more bioavailable.

- If you're using a blender, add a half-cup of water to your recipe, blend the herbs up with everything else, chop the bigger stuff up incredibly finely, and add more water as needed to get your blender going. Serve chilled!

Belly-Booster Juice

This juice is designed to help heal your digestive system. Whether it's always had trouble or been feeling wonky only recently, a daily dose of this drink might be exactly what you need to heal!

This recipe needs less than 5 minutes of prep to be ready! It will make up to 4 helpings, depending on how much you can drink.

What to Use:

- Pineapple (one-third of a whole pineapple)
- Carrot (1 large-sized)
- Lemon (0.5 lemon with rind)
- Mint (0.5 packed cup fresh herb, washed well)
- Ginger (half-inch of root)
- Apple Cider Vinegar (1 tablespoon stirred in at the end)
- 1 juicer (or 1 blender could work, too)

What to Do:

- If you have a juicer, add everything into your juicer, process, and drink as soon as possible. Make sure to put your mint greens in between two big pieces of something else otherwise they might not be able to be fully juiced. Stir in the ACV at the end to get another boost of belly-treating power in this drink!

- If you're using a blender, add a half-cup of water to your recipe, cut everything up much smaller, and add more water as needed to get your blender going. Serve chilled!

Steaming & Freezing Herbs – Decoctions, Teas & Treats

Taking things almost to the point of boil or way beyond the point of chill, this section looks at a couple additional ways to approach your herbal healing. Some snacks are incorporated alongside healing teas and herbal decoctions. You should find your every craving suited in this section, and you might even find yourself inspired to try a few new things along the same veins as what's presented in the following pages. Never be afraid to get creative, and as always (unless you're making tea!), stay as fresh with those herbs as you can.

DIY Herbal Decoctions

Decoctions are a huge part of herbal healing, but they work more on the subtle realms of energy rather than the more obvious. By extracting the essence of the herb in a bowl of water with the power of the light of the sun, you can pull out the subtle energies of the plant that help it enact healing. Then, by preserving this extraction with just a dash of alcohol, you can keep it for months, if not years, and use that healing in small doses each day. Give it a try, and you might be surprised at what happens.

This recipe needs a minute of prep and about a day of "cooking." It will make several helpings for the future.

What to Use:

- Water (1 gallon, purified)
- Vodka (1 dash, for preservation)
- Herbs (whatever herbs you choose, although, use only one per decoction)
- The sun!
- 1 large glass jar or 1 large glass bowl

What to Do:

- Take your large glass jar or bowl and pour the water into it. Take the jar or bowl and set it outside where it will receive ample sunlight.

- Choose the herb you want to decoct and grab a few sprigs of it in its fresh form. Add the herb to the water.
- Let the water infuse with the herb's energy for up to a full day's worth of sunlight and then take the herbs out of your water and discard them. Pour all the liquid back into the gallon water container.
- In that gallon container, add a dash of vodka (or another clear liquor) as a preservative and seal.
- Take one swig of the water each day or add drops to your standard water bottle. Do not drink too quickly to be able to fully enjoy the subtle effects this decoction has on your health.

Hawthorne Tea for Heart Health

Hawthorne tea promotes the health of your heart, your blood, and your circulatory system. It prevents cardiovascular diseases when taken regularly, and it can lower blood pressure, easing hypertension as well as anxiety and stress responses.

This recipe needs a minute of prep and 10 minutes of cooking. It will make 1 helping.

What to Use:

- Hawthorne Leaves or Hawthorne Flower Petals (1.5 tablespoons of the *dried* herbs)
- Water (1.5 cups)
- 1 small-sized pot
- 1 tea ball (if you have it)
- 1 coffee mug

What to Do:

- On medium heat, bring your water to a low boil.
- Gather your dried herbs and put them into your tea ball or simply add them to the water.
- Let the tea roll on a low boil for just a second after the herbs are added, then

turn the heat completely off to allow the tea to steep.

- After 5-10 minutes of steeping, strain out the herbs from the water or just remove your tea ball. Serve hot.

Chamomile Ginger Tea for Calming

Together, chamomile and ginger calm the body, mind, and soul. They help with an upset stomach as well as an upset mind and can reduce anxiety as well as nausea. It can even calm you so much that it helps with sleep issues. Overall, this tea is great for your immune system, your pain response, and your stress response. You're sure to love it.

This recipe needs 2 minutes of prep and 10 minutes of cooking. It will make 1 helping.

What to Use:

- Chamomile Leaves or Chamomile Flower Petals (1 tablespoon of the *dried* herbs)
- Ginger (1 half-inch of the root, sliced)
- Water (1.5 cups)
- 1 small-sized pot
- 1 tea ball (if you have it)
- 1 coffee mug

What to Do:

- On medium heat, bring your water to a low boil.
- Gather your dried herbs and put them into your tea ball or simply add them to the

water. Slice the ginger and put it into the pot as well.

- Let the tea roll on a low boil for just a second after the herbs are added, then turn the heat completely off to allow the tea to steep.
- After 5-10 minutes of steeping, strain out the herbs from the water or just remove your tea ball. Serve hot.

Valerian Thyme Tea for Longevity

Valerian and thyme work together to lessen the intensity of day-to-day life. If you're often overtired or stressed beyond belief – may be so stressed that you have issues with ulcers or seizures. Valerian will help you feel rested in even the most trying times, while thyme works to rebuild brain cells and refuses to let your respiration fall out of tip-top shape.

This recipe needs a minute of prep and 10 minutes of cooking. It will make 1 helping.

What to Use:

- Valerian Leaves (1 tablespoon of the *dried* herbs)
- Thyme (0.5 tablespoon of the dried herbs or 2 sprigs fresh herb)
- Water (1.5 cups)
- 1 small-sized pot
- 1 tea ball (if you have it)
- 1 coffee mug

What to Do:

- On medium heat, bring your water to a low boil.
- Gather your dried herbs and put them into your tea ball or simply add them to the water.

- Let the tea roll on a low boil for just a second after the herbs are added, then turn the heat completely off to allow the tea to steep.
- After 5-10 minutes of steeping, strain out the herbs from the water or just remove your tea ball. Serve hot.

Echinacea Tea with Lemon for the Cold & Flu Season

As one of the best cold & flu season herbs, echinacea works constantly to jolt your immune system and protect against infections. If you have nasal congestion issues or infections related to your skin or inner body, this tea would be perfect for you. Avoid this tea if you're pregnant, but otherwise, it's perfect to flush any flu symptom or hint of infection.

This recipe needs 2 minutes of prep and 10 minutes of cooking. It will make 1 helping.

What to Use:

- Echinacea Tea (1.5 tablespoons of the *dried* herbs)
- Lemon (0.5 lemon, juiced)
- Honey or Vegan Sweetener (0.5 teaspoon)
- Water (1.5 cups)
- 1 small-sized pot
- 1 tea ball (if you have it)
- 1 coffee mug

- On medium heat, bring your water to a low boil.
- Gather your dried herbs and put them into your tea ball or simply add them to the water.
- Let the tea roll on a low boil for just a second after the herbs are added, then turn the heat completely off to allow the tea to steep.
- After 5-10 minutes of steeping, strain out the herbs from the water or just remove your tea ball. Add the lemon juice and honey last. Serve hot.

Peppermint Dandelion Tea for Detox

Together, peppermint and dandelion are the dream-team of digestion herbs. Peppermint soothes an upset stomach and relieves digestive inflammation, while dandelion improves the function of the liver, kidneys, and stomach. With this tea, your body will be completely flushed of toxins as long as you drink a cup daily! Try harvesting dandelions from your yard in summer (as long as you don't spray your yard with pesticides or herbicides) and dry them to have this tea all throughout the year!

This recipe needs 0 minutes of prep and 10 minutes of cooking. It will make 1 helping.

What to Use:

- Peppermint Leaves (1 tablespoon of the *dried* herbs)
- Dandelion Flowers (1 tablespoon of *dried* flowers)
- Water (1.5 cups)
- 1 small-sized pot
- 1 tea ball (if you have it)
- 1 coffee mug

What to Do:

- On medium heat, bring your water to a low boil.
- Gather your dried herbs and put them into your tea ball or simply add them to the water.
- Let the tea roll on a low boil for just a second after the herbs are added, then turn the heat completely off to allow the tea to steep.
- After 5-10 minutes of steeping, strain out the herbs from the water or just remove your tea ball. Serve hot.

Traditional Golden Milk

This old-world Indian drink has been used for centuries because of its healing abilities. It applies lemon, ginger, and turmeric in healing work together with some black pepper to make the effects fully bioavailable! It's the new winter drink you've been craving that will boost your energy and vitality on even the darkest of days.

This recipe needs 5 minutes of prep and 20 minutes of cooking. It will make 2 helpings.

What to Use:

- Unsweetened Non-Dairy Milk or Regular Milk (1.5 cups)
- Cinnamon Stick (1 three-inch stick)
- Turmeric (1 inch-long piece of root, unpeeled & sliced thinly OR 0.5 teaspoon *dried* turmeric)
- Ginger (1 half-inch piece of root, unpeeled & sliced thinly)
- Honey or Probiotic Vegan Sweetener (1 tablespoon)
- Coconut Oil (1 tablespoon)
- Black Peppercorns (0.25 teaspoon whole peppercorns)
- Water (1 cup)
- Cinnamon (ground & dried herb, for garnish)

- 1 small-sized pot
- 2 coffee mugs

What to Do:

- Whisk together all ingredients except ground cinnamon in a small pot. On medium-high heat, bring to low boil.
- Once boil is achieved, turn down to simmer for 10 minutes until all flavors are well-combined.
- Strain through a colander, sieve, or cheesecloth to catch any peppercorns or fibers from the roots. Serve in coffee mugs with a dash of cinnamon.

Garam Masala Snacks

This snack *can* be made a multitude of different ways. In specific, this recipe delineates a process of making raw, flavored nut snacks with a food dehydrator, but you could always turn on the oven to 350 degrees F and cook in increments of 5 minutes, stirring after each segment of time and finishing when the nuts begin to crackle and they're only lightly browned (around 20 minutes, total).

Garam Masala Snacks require anywhere from 15 minutes to 8 hours of prep and anywhere from 20 minutes to 6 hours of cooking. The recipe will make 8 helpings.

What to Use:

- Nuts (2 cups of any one of the following or a mixture between a few: cashews, almonds, pecans, or walnuts)
- Water (4 cups)
- Garam Masala (2.5 tablespoons):
    - Cumin (4 parts; ground & dried seed)
    - Coriander (2 parts; ground & dried seed)
    - Cardamom (2 parts; ground & dried seed)
    - Black Pepper (2 parts)

o   Cinnamon (1 part; ground herb)
o   Cloves (1 part; ground herb)
- Salt (0.5 teaspoon)
- 1 medium-sized bowl
- 1 food dehydrator (or 1 baking sheet for cooking in the oven, if you so choose)

What to Do:

- Soak your nuts in the 4 cups of water for at least 4 hours and no longer than 8 hours. In the middle of your time, stir everything up and maybe add a splash more water if your nuts have soaked up a lot.
- When the time is up, rinse them, drain them, and pour them into your bowl. Sprinkle in garam masala and salt; stir till completely coated.
- Grab your dehydrator and set out the nuts on two separate trays. One tray will work if your dehydrator only has space for one. Turn the temperature to 105 degrees F and dehydrate for up to 8 hours.
- Enjoy! These tasty snacks will keep for up to two weeks.

Sweet & Spicy Nuts

This recipe is easy and fast. It only takes about a minute of actual "cooking" before you're ready to munch. If you're interested and able, you can always dehydrate your nuts for up to 6 hours on 105 degrees F and enjoy them that way as well. It just depends how sticky you want to get and how long you're able to wait!

This recipe needs less than 15 minutes of prep and less than 5 minutes of "cooking." It will make 4 helpings.

What to Use:

- Nuts (2 cups of any one of the following or a mixture between a few: cashews, almonds, pecans, or walnuts – or others! Get creative!)
- Dates (0.5 cup, pitted OR 0.5 cup maple syrup or honey)
- Water (*if using dates* 0.5 cup)
- Salt (0.5 teaspoon)
- Cayenne Pepper (0.25 teaspoon)
- Cardamom (0.5 teaspoon, dried & ground seed)
- Nutmeg (0.25 teaspoon)
- 1 small-sized bowl
- 1 medium-sized bowl

What to Do:

- If you're using dates, pit them and soak them in water in your small-sized bowl for around 10 minutes. When that's done, mash the dates into the water with the back of a fork until you've made a sort of date paste.
- In the medium-sized bowl, mix together the sweetener, salt, pepper, cardamom, and nutmeg. Stir in your nuts until completely coated by your topping and eat right away...as if you could stop yourself!

DIY "Dolmas"!

In this variation of traditional dolmas, we'll substitute the grape leaf for a collard green, but you can always go the original way instead of as you please! To make things simpler for yourself, go with the collards. They're great for you and they may not be an herb, but they are an easily-accessibly vehicle for the goodness that hides inside.

This recipe needs 15 minutes of prep and 5 minutes of "cooking." It will make 4 helpings.

What to Use:

- Brown Rice (1 cup, precooked)
- Sundried Tomatoes (0.75 cup, sliced)
- Water (1 cup)
- Dill (0.25 cup fresh herb, chopped; use 1.5 tablespoons if dried herb)
- Kalamata Olives (2 tablespoons, pitted & sliced)
- Pine Nuts (0.5 cup)
- Extra Virgin Olive Oil (2 tablespoons)
- Salt (to taste)
- Collard Greens (2 + large, broad leaves destemmed)
- 1 medium-sized bowl

- In your medium sized bowl, mix together your sundried tomatoes and water. Let sit for 10 minutes so that the tomatoes soften nicely. Drain out the water from the bowl.
- Add in your rice, nuts, raisins, oil, salt, and fresh or dried dill. Stir together until well-combined.
- Grab your collard green. If the leaf itself is broader than 6 inches even after being destemmed, cut it in half vertically and then in half horizontally so that you have four pieces.
- Put a quarter of the filling into each quarter and wrap it as best you can. If you need to use the leaf as more of a "taco shell," do it that way instead! You're sure to love this flavor!

Herbal Coconut Chutney

This dish is more of a topping or side than an entrée, but it's flavor and health impact are equally dynamic. You can find young coconuts at many supermarkets as well as health food stores, so don't be worried about finding coconut meat. I assure you, it'll be easier than you think! The tricky part is getting that coconut meat *out* of its shell. Regardless, this recipe is worth the work since it's full of cancer-fighting powers and inflammation-flushing potential.

This recipe needs 15 minutes of prep (sometimes opening coconuts is hard work!) and 5 minutes of "cooking." It will make 4 helpings.

What to Use:

- Coconut Meat (extracted from 2-3 coconuts; Thai baby coconuts preferred)
  - ** Look up a video on how to do this extraction safely! **
  - Basically, you'll need to cut a hole into the top of the coconut if there isn't one there already. Don't let children attempt this feat and try to keep your hands off the coconut itself while you wield your knife because you can very easily get in

> your own way to a problematic extent.
>
> o Grab a cutting board and a large knife. Cut three slits into the top of the coconut that all touch one another and form the shape of a triangle.
> o Drink out the coconut water with a straw if you want or just drain it out.
> o Take a meat cleaver if you have one or the biggest knife you have and aim it right at the middle of your coconut now, not in a stabbing motion, but so that the blade comes down to push its way through the exact middle of the coconut, halving it.
> o Scoop out the fleshy bits from inside the coconut shell with a spoon – this "meat" is exactly what you're looking for!

- Lemon (0.5, juiced)
- Garlic (1 clove, minced)
- Thai Red Chili Pepper (1 small-sized, diced)
- Cilantro (0.5 cup, fresh leaves, chopped finely)
- Yellow Onion (0.25 cup, chopped finely)

- Salt (0.5 teaspoon)
- 1 blender
- 1 medium-sized bowl

What to Do:

- Start by taking a quarter-cup of your coconut meat and adding it to the blender with your lemon juice. Blend together until smooth.
- Pour into your bowl and then add the remaining "meat," the minced garlic, and the finely chopped chili, cilantro, and onion. Sprinkle in the salt and mix well.
- Serve as desired or eat alone proudly!

Apple Martini Popsicle

This refreshing popsicle is not only perfect for summer days, but it's perfect in its healing capacity for *any* day! If you want, substitute the soda for champagne or liquor to give a bit of a bite to your healing frozen snack.

This recipe needs 15 minutes of prep and several hours of freezing. It will make up to 8 helpings.

What to Use:

- Cucumber (1, peeled & seeded)
- Apple (2 large-sized, peeled & seeded)
- Mint (a packed half-cup of fresh leaves)
- Basil (1 sprig fresh herb)
- Lime (2, juiced & zested)
- 7-UP or Sprite or Carbonated Water (2.5 cups)
- *if using carbonated water* Syrup (0.5 tablespoon)
- *if using carbonated water* Lemon Juice (2 tablespoons)
- 1 or 2 popsicle racks – enough for 8-10 popsicles

What to Do:

- Put everything in the blender and pulse until completely smooth.
- Pour into the popsicle racks and freeze for at least 3 hours before serving.
- Enjoy!

Conclusion

As you come to the end of your experience with the *Herbal Medicine Cooker*, for now, you should feel prepared as you decide to venture forward. You should know a good number of herbs and their medicinal uses, and you should also have a sense of what recipes to use for your goals. Furthermore, you should feel confident that you can use a diet infused with herbs to help yourself lose that weight or finally get better. If you're not convinced, do a little more research and then come back to this book. The opportunity *Herbal Medicine Cooker* offers of your healing will remain – eagerly waiting for your return.

Whether this is the first, third, fiftieth, or thousandth step on the path of herbal medicine, you should feel ready to move forward once more through the information provided in these pages. All you have to do now is gather the ingredients, find yourself a fresh herb connection, and get creative! You may even soon find yourself inspired to grow herbs yourself, as you can, for your connection with these herbs is only just beginning. You'll surely be surprised where it takes you.

If you noticed an herb from chapter 2 that wasn't included in any of these recipes, feel free to expand your search into the wide world of recipes that exists elsewhere. You can always take the table from that chapter to guide your pursuit of the perfect recipe to respond to your disease or ailment, whether it's weak ankles, a broken bone, or almost anything you could imagine.

Herbal medicine is both timeless and *timely*. Humans have been so largely out of touch with the health of our surrounding environments that we've lost many of the plants our ancestors used for healing, and we're also so out of touch with the abilities of plants in general that we've supplanted herbal healing for almost anything *but*. As true as it is that this curative technique has existed across the ages, it is also true that we need it now more than ever, after having lost so much of that original knowledge. This book – and your download of it – works against that loss; they work toward health instead, toward growth, life, and creativity.

Congratulations on being a part of something so beautiful.

This book belongs to a series of books about herbal medicine and how to use it to improve our life. For more information, visit:

www.db-publishing.com